The Plant-Based Guide to Healthy Cooking

Delicious Plant-Based Recipes for Good Health

Ben Goleman

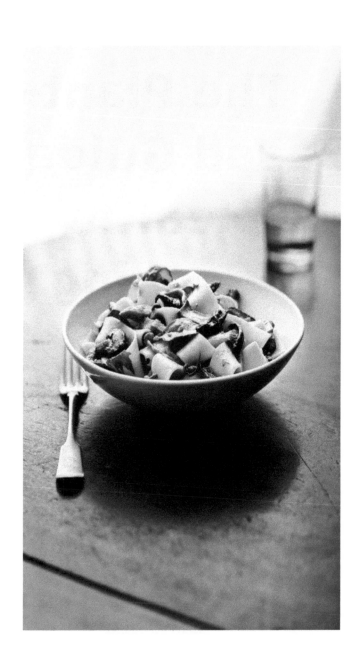

1

engaging in the rendering of legal, financial, medical or professional advice. The content within this book has been derived from various sources. Please consult a licensed professional before attempting any techniques outlined in this book.

By reading this document, the reader agrees that under no circumstances is the author responsible for any losses, direct or indirect, which are incurred as a result of the use of information contained within this document, including, but not limited to, — errors, omissions, or inaccuracies.

Table of Contents

Last-minute Macaroons

Servings: 10

Cooking Time: 15 Minutes

Ingredients:

- 3 cups coconut flakes, sweetened
- 9 ounces canned coconut milk, sweetened
- 1 teaspoon ground anise
- 1 teaspoon vanilla extract

Directions:

1. Begin by preheating your oven to 325 degrees F. Line the cookie sheets with parchment paper.

2. Thoroughly combine all the ingredients until everything is well incorporated.

3. Use a cookie scoop to drop mounds of the batter onto the prepared cookie sheets.

4. Bake for about 11 minutes until they are lightly browned. Bon appétit!

Nutrition Info: Per Serving: Calories: 125; Fat: 7.2g; Carbs: 14.3g; Protein: 1.1g

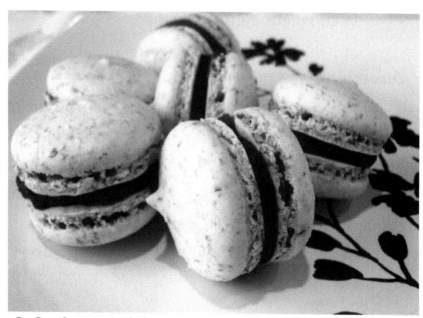

Apple & Cashew Quiche

Servings: 6

Cooking Time: 55 Minutes

Ingredients:

- 5 apples, peeled and cut into slices
- ½ cup pure maple syrup
- 1 tbsp fresh orange juice
- 1 tsp ground cinnamon
- ½ cup whole-grain flour
- ½ cup old-fashioned oats
- ½ cup finely chopped cashew
- ⅔ cup pure date sugar
- ½ cup plant butter, softened

Directions:

1. Preheat oven to 360 F. Place apples in a greased baking pan. Stir in maple syrup and orange juice. Sprinkle with ½ tsp of cinnamon. In a bowl, combine the flour, oats, cashew, sugar, and remaining cinnamon. Blend in the butter until the mixture crumbs. Pour over the apples and bake for 45 minutes.

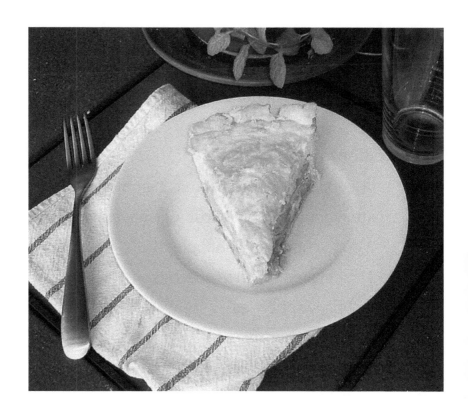

Minty Fruit Salad

Servings: 4

Cooking Time: 5 Minutes

Ingredients:

- ¼ cup lemon juice (about 2 small lemons)
- 4teaspoons maple syrup or agave syrup
- 2 cups chopped pineapple
- 2 cups chopped strawberries
- 2 cups raspberries
- 1 cup blueberries
- 8 fresh mint leaves

Directions:

1. Preparing the Ingredients

2. Beginning with 1 mason jar, add the ingredients in this order: 1 tablespoon of lemon juice, 1 teaspoon of maple syrup, ½ cup of pineapple, ½ cup of strawberries, ½ cup of raspberries, ¼ cup of blueberries, and 2 mint leaves.

3. Finish and Serve

4. Repeat to fill 3 more jars. Close the jars tightly with lids.

5. Place the airtight jars in the refrigerator for up to 3 days.

Nutrition Info: Per Serving: Calories: 138; Fat: 1g; Protein: 2g; Carbohydrates: 34g; Fiber: 8g; Sugar: 22g;

Sodium: 6mg

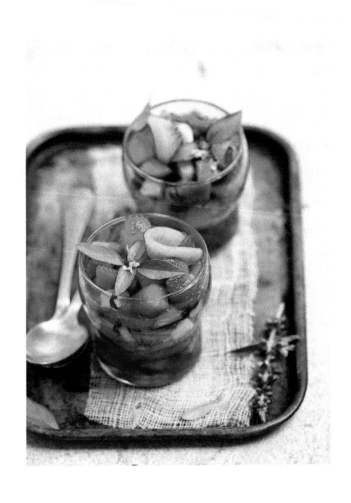

Holiday Pecan Tart

Servings: 4

Cooking Time: 50 Minutes

Ingredients:

- 4 tbsp flax seed powder
- 1/3 cup whole-wheat flour
- ½ tsp salt
- ¼ cup cold plant butter, crumbled
- 3 tbsp pure malt syrup
- 3 tbsp flax seed powder + 9 tbsp water
- 2 cups toasted pecans, chopped
- 1 cup light corn syrup
- ½ cup pure date sugar
- 1 tbsp pure pomegranate molasses
- 4 tbsp plant butter, melted
- ½ tsp salt
- 2 tsp vanilla extract

Directions:

1.   Preheat the oven to 350 F. In a bowl, mix the flax seed powder with tbsp water and allow thickening for 5 minutes. Do this for the filling's flax

egg too in a separate bowl. In a large bowl, combine flour and salt.

Add in plant butter and whisk until crumbly. Pour in the crust's flax egg and maple syrup and mix until smooth dough forms. Flatten the dough on a flat surface, cover with plastic wrap, and refrigerate for 1 hour. Dust a working surface with flour, remove the dough onto the surface, and using a rolling pin, flatten the dough into a 1-inch diameter circle. Lay the dough on a greased pie pan and press to fit the shape of the pan. Trim the edges of the pan. Lay a parchment paper on the dough, pour on some baking beans and bake for 20 minutes. Remove the pan, pour out the baking beans, and allow cooling.

2.   In a bowl, mix the filling's flax egg, pecans, corn syrup, date sugar, pomegranate molasses, plant butter, salt, and vanilla. Pour and spread the mixture on the piecrust. Bake further for minutes or until the filling sets. Remove from the oven, decorate with more pecans, slice, and cool. Slice and serve.

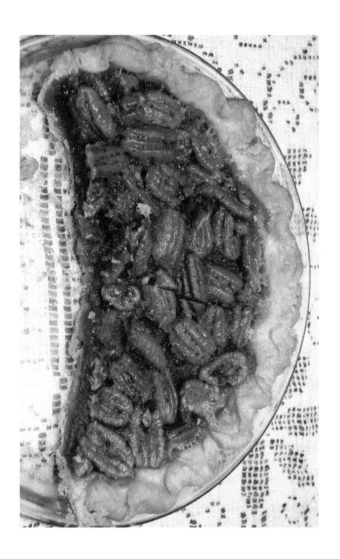

Pressure Cooker Apple Cupcakes

Servings: 4

Cooking Time: 25 Minutes

Ingredients:

- 1 cup canned applesauce
- 1 cup non-dairy milk
- 6 tbsp maple syrup + for sprinkling
- ¼ cup spelt flour
- ½ tsp apple pie spice
- A pinch of salt

Directions:

1. In a bowl, combine the applesauce, milk, maple syrup, flour, apple pie spice, and salt. Scoop into 4 heat-proof ramekins. Drizzle with more syrup.

2. Pour 1 cup of water in the IP and fit in a trivet. Place the ramekins on the trivet. Lock lid in place; set the time to 6 minutes on High. Once ready, perform a quick pressure release. Unlock the lid and let cool for a few minutes take out the ramekins. Allow to cool for 10 minutes and serve.

Chocolate Mousse

Servings: 2

Cooking Time: 0 Minute

Ingredients:

- 6 drops liquid stevia extract
- ½ t. cinnamon
- 3 tbsp. cocoa powder, unsweetened
- 1 c. coconut milk

Directions:

1. On the day before, place the coconut milk into the refrigerator overnight.

2. Remove the coconut milk from the refrigerator; it should be very thick.

3. Whisk in cocoa powder with an electric mixer.

4. Add stevia and cinnamon and whip until combined.

5. Place in individual bowls and serve and enjoy.

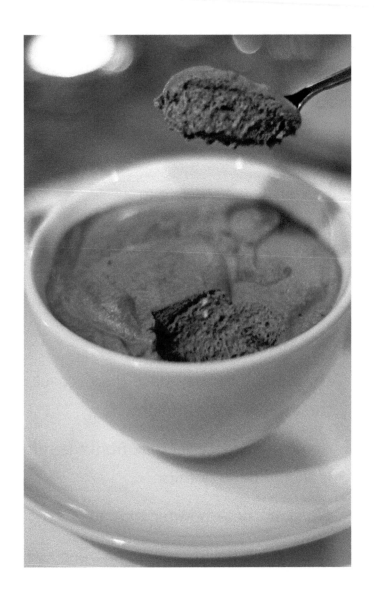

Almond-date Energy Bites

Servings: 24

Cooking Time: 15 Minutes

Ingredients:

- 1 cup dates, pitted
- 1 cup unsweetened shredded coconut
- ¼ cup chia seeds
- ¾ cup ground almonds
- ¼ cup cocoa nibs, or non-dairy chocolate chips

Directions:

1. Preparing the Ingredients.

2. Purée everything in a food processor until crumbly and sticking together, pushing down the sides whenever necessary to keep it blending. If you don't have a food processor, you can mash soft Medjool dates. But if you're using harder baking dates, you'll have to soak them, then try to purée them in a blender.

3. Finish and Serve

4.   Form the mix into 2balls and place them on a baking sheet lined with parchment or waxed paper. Put in the fridge to set for about 15 minutes. Use the softest dates you can find. Medjool dates are the best for this purpose. The hard dates you see in the baking aisle of your supermarket are going to take a long time to blend up. If you use those, try soaking them in water for at least an hour before you start, and then start draining.

Nutrition Info: Per Serving: (1 bite) Calories 152; Total fat: 11g; Carbs: 13g; Fiber: 5g; Protein: 3g

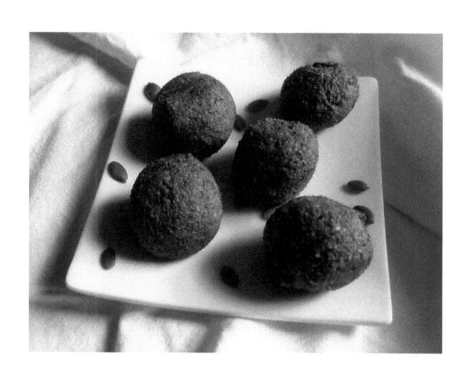

Peach-mango Crumble (pressure Cooker)

Servings: 4-6

Cooking Time: 21 Minutes

Ingredients:

- 3 cups chopped fresh or frozen peaches
- 3 cups chopped fresh or frozen mangos
- 4 tablespoons unrefined sugar or pure maple syrup, divided
- 1 cup gluten-free rolled oats
- ½ cup shredded coconut, sweetened or unsweetened
- 2 tablespoons coconut oil or vegan margarine

Directions:

1. Preparing the Ingredients. In a 6- to 7-inch round baking dish, toss together the peaches, mangos, and 2 tablespoons of sugar. In a food processor, combine the oats, coconut, coconut oil, and remaining 2 tablespoons of sugar. Pulse until combined. (If you use maple syrup, you'll need less coconut oil. Start with just the syrup and add oil if the mixture isn't sticking together.) Sprinkle the oat mixture over the fruit mixture.

2. Cover the dish with aluminum foil. Put a trivet in the bottom of your electric pressure cooker's cooking pot and pour in a cup or two of water. Using a foil sling or silicone helper handles, lower the pan onto the trivet.

3. High pressure for 6 minutes. Close and lock the lid, and select High Pressure for 6 minutes.

4. Pressure Release. Once the cook time is complete, quick release the pressure. Unlock and remove the lid.

5. Let cool for a few minutes before carefully lifting out the dish with oven mitts or tongs. Scoop out portions to serve.

Nutrition Info: Per Serving: Calories: 321; Total fat:

18g; Protein: 4g; Sodium: 2mg; Fiber: 7g

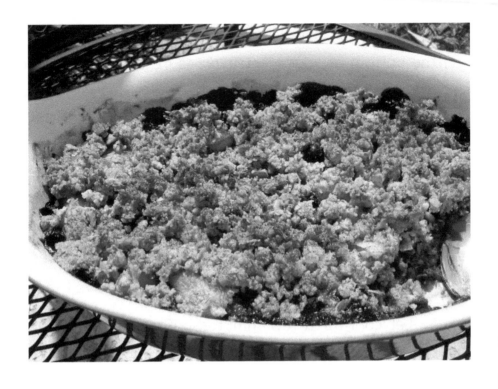

Lime Avocado Ice Cream

Servings: 4

Cooking Time: 10 Minutes

Ingredients:

- 2 large avocados, pitted
- Juice and zest of 3 limes • 1/3 cup erythritol
- 1 ¾ cups coconut cream
- ¼ tsp vanilla extract

Directions:

1. In a blender, combine the avocado pulp, lime juice and zest, erythritol, coconut cream, and vanilla extract. Process until the mixture is smooth. Pour the mixture into your ice cream maker and freeze based on the manufacturer's instructions. When ready, remove and scoop the ice cream into bowls. Serve immediately.

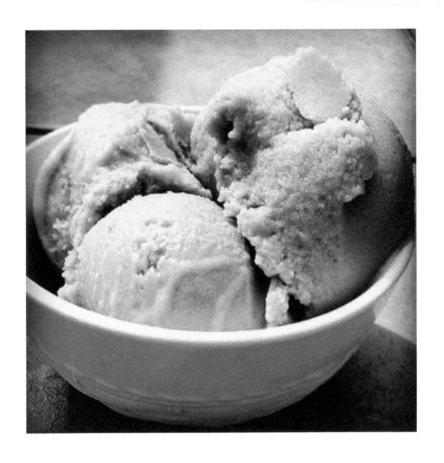

Walnut Chocolate Squares

Servings: 6

Cooking Time: 10 Minutes

Ingredients:

- 3½ oz dairy-free dark chocolate
- 4 tbsp plant butter
- 1 pinch salt
- ¼ cup walnut butter
- ½ tsp vanilla extract
- ¼ cup chopped walnuts to garnish

Directions:

1. Pour the chocolate and plant butter in a safe microwave bowl and melt in the microwave for about to 2 minutes. Remove the bowl from the microwave and mix in the salt, walnut butter, and vanilla.

2. Grease a small baking sheet with cooking spray and line with parchment paper. Pour in the batter and use a spatula to spread out into a 4 x 6-inch rectangle. Top with the chopped walnuts and chill in the refrigerator. Once set, cut into 1 x 1-inch squares. Serve while firming.

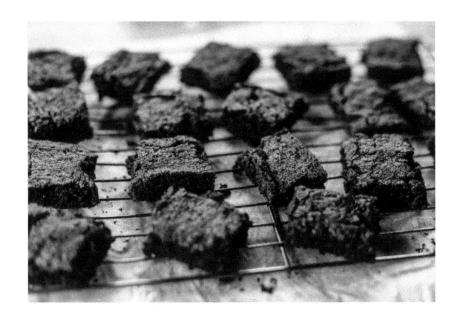

Vegetable Mushroom Side Dish

Servings: 4

Cooking Time: 60 Minutes

Ingredients:

- 2 tbsp plant butter
- 1 large onion, diced
- 1 cup celery, diced
- ½ cup carrots, diced
- ½ tsp dried marjoram
- 1 tsp dried basil
- 2 cups chopped cremini mushrooms
- 1 cup vegetable broth
- ¼ cup chopped fresh parsley
- 1 medium whole-grain bread loaf, cubed

Directions:

1. Melt the butter in large skillet and sauté the onion, celery, mushrooms, and carrots until softened, 5 minutes.

2. Mix in the marjoram, basil, and season with salt and black pepper.

3. Pour in the vegetable broth and mix in the parsley and bread. Cook until the broth reduces by half, 10 minutes.

4. Pour the mixture into a baking dish and cover with foil. Bake in the oven at 375 F for 30 minutes.

5. Uncover and bake further for 30 minutes or until golden brown on top and the liquid absorbs.

6. Remove the dish from the oven and serve the stuffing.

Chocolate Macaroons

Servings: 8

Cooking Time: 15 Minutes

Ingredients:

- 1 cup unsweetened shredded coconut
- 2 tablespoons cocoa powder
- ⅔ cup coconut milk
- ¼ cup agave
- pinch of sea salt

Directions:

1. Preparing the Ingredients.

2. Preheat the oven to 350°F. Line a baking sheet with parchment paper. In a medium saucepan, cook all the ingredients over medium-high heat until a firm dough is formed. Scoop the dough into balls and place on the baking sheet.

3. Bake

4. Bake for 15 minutes, remove from the oven, and let it cool on the baking sheet. Serve cooled macaroons.

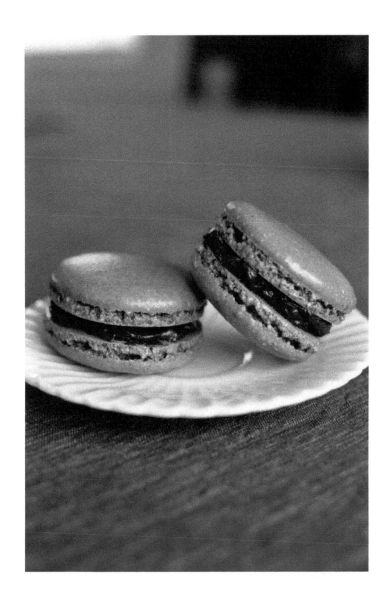

Mixed Berry Yogurt Ice Pops

Servings: 6

Cooking Time: 5 Minutes

Ingredients:

- 2/3 cup avocado, halved and pitted
- 2/3 cup frozen berries, thawed
- 1 cup dairy-free yogurt
- ½ cup coconut cream
- 1 tsp vanilla extract

Directions:

1. Pour the avocado pulp, berries, dairy-free yogurt, coconut cream, and vanilla extract. Process until smooth. Pour into ice pop sleeves and freeze for 8 or more hours.

Enjoy the ice pops when ready.

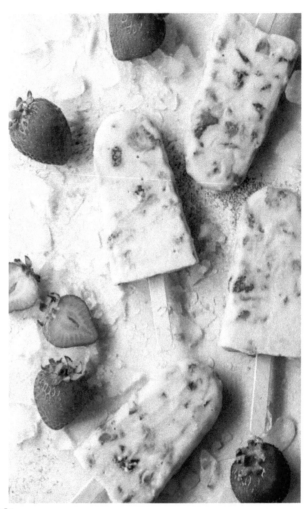

Risotto Bites

Servings: 12

Cooking Time: 20 Minutes

Ingredients:

- ½ cup panko bread crumbs
- 1 teaspoon paprika

- 1 teaspoon chipotle powder or ground cayenne pepper
- 1½ cups cold Green Pea Risotto
- Nonstick cooking spray

Directions:

1. Preparing the Ingredients.

2. Preheat the oven to 4ºF.

3. Line a baking sheet with parchment paper.

4. On a large plate, combine the panko, paprika, and chipotle powder. Set aside.

5. Roll 2 tablespoons of the risotto into a ball.

6. Gently roll in the bread crumbs, and place on the prepared baking sheet. Repeat to make a total of 12 balls.

7. Spritz the tops of the risotto bites with nonstick cooking spray and bake for 15 to 20 minutes, until they begin to brown. Cool completely before storing in a large airtight container in a single layer (add a piece of parchment paper for a second layer) or in a plastic freezer bag.

Nutrition Info: Calories: 100; Fat: 2g; Protein: 6g; Carbohydrates: 17g; Fiber: 5g; Sugar: 2g; Sodium: 165 mg

Brownie Bites

Servings: 8

Cooking Time: 0 Minutes

Ingredients:

- ¾ cup blanched almond flour
- ¾ cup cacao powder
- 2 tablespoons ground flaxseed
- ½ cup unsweetened vegan mini chocolate chips
- ¾ cup creamy almond butter, melted
- ¼ cup pure maple syrup
- 1 teaspoon pure vanilla extract

Directions:

1. In a large bowl, mix together the almond flour, cocoa powder, flaxseed, and chocolate chips.

2. Add the almond butter, maple syrup, and vanilla extract, and gently stir to combine.

3. Using a sturdy spatula, stir and fold together until well incorporated.

4. With your hands, make equal-sized balls from mixture.

5. Arrange the balls onto a parchment paper-lined baking sheet in a single layer.

6. Refrigerate to set for about 15 minutes before serving.

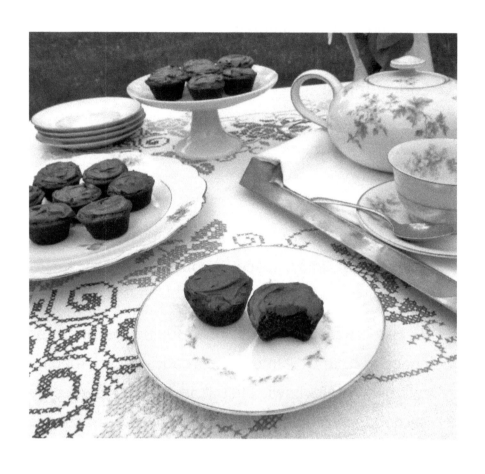

Fudge

Servings: 18

Cooking Time: 5 Minutes

Ingredients:

- 1 cup vegan chocolate chips
- ½ cup soy milk

Directions:

1. Line an 8-inch portion skillet with wax paper. Set aside. Clear some space in your refrigerator for this dish as you will need it later.

2. Melt chocolate chips in a double boiler or add chocolate and almond spread to a medium, microwavesafe bowl. Melt it in the microwave in - second increments until chocolate melts. In between each 20second burst, stir the chocolate until it is smooth.

3. Empty the melted chocolate mixture into the lined skillet. Tap the sides of the skillet to make sure the mixture spreads into an even layer. Alternatively, use a spoon to make swirls on top.

4. Move skillet to the refrigerator until it is firm. Remove the skillet from the refrigerator and cut fudge into 18 squares.

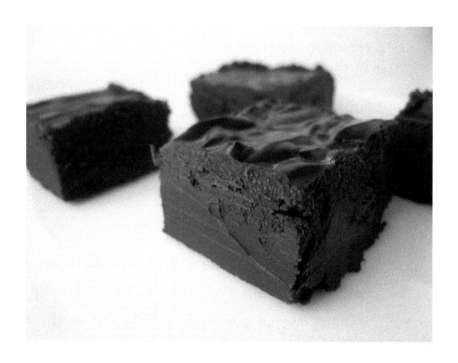

Sesame

Servings: 3

Cooking Time: 12 Minutes

Ingredients:

- ¾ cup vegan margarine, softened
- ½ cup light brown sugar
- 1 teaspoon pure vanilla extract
- 2 tablespoons pure maple syrup
- ¼ teaspoon salt
- 2 cups whole-grain flour
- ¾ cup sesame seeds, lightly toasted

Directions:

1. Preparing the Ingredients

2. In a large bowl, cream together the margarine and sugar until light and fluffy. Blend in the vanilla, maple syrup, and salt. Stir in the flour and sesame seeds and mix well.

3. Roll the dough into a cylinder about 2 inches in diameter. Wrap it in plastic wrap and refrigerate for 1 hour or longer. Preheat the oven to 5°F.

4. Slice the cookie dough into 1/8-inch-thick rounds and arrange on an ungreased baking sheet about 2 inches apart.

5. Bake

6. Bake until light brown for about 12 minutes. When completely cool, store in an airtight container.

Tacos

Servings: 4

Cooking Time: 30 Minutes

Ingredients:

- 6 Taco Shells
- For the slaw:
- 1 cup Red Cabbage, shredded
- 3 Scallions, chopped
- 1 cup Green Cabbage, shredded
- 1 cup Carrots, sliced
- For the dressing:
- 1 tbsp. Sriracha
- ¼ cup Apple Cider Vinegar
- ¼ tsp. Salt
- 2 tbsp. Sesame Oil
- 1 tbsp. Dijon Mustard
- 1 tbsp. Lime Juice
- ½ tbsp. Tamari
- 1 tbsp. Maple Syrup
- ¼ tsp. Salt

Directions:

1. To start with, make the dressing, whisk all the ingredients in a small bowl until mixed well.

2. Next, combine the slaw ingredients in another bowl and toss well.

3. Finally, take a taco shell and place the slaw in it.

4. Serve and enjoy

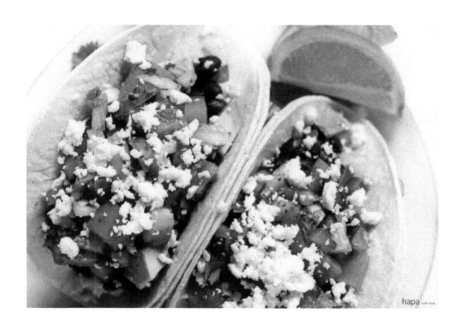

Kale Chips 2

Servings: 10

Cooking Time: 1 Hour 30 Minutes

Ingredients:

* ½ tsp. Smoked Paprika
* 2 bunches of Curly Kale
* 1 tsp. Garlic Powder
* ½ cup Nutritional Yeast
* 2 cups Cashew, soaked for 2 hours
* 1 tsp. Salt
* ½ cup Nutritional Yeast

Directions:

1. To make these tasty, healthy chips place the kale in a large mixing bowl.

2. Now, combine all the remaining ingredients in the high-speed blender and blend for 1 minute or until smooth.

3. Next, pour this dressing over the kale chips and mix well with your hands.

4. Then, preheat your oven to 225 ° F or 107 °C.

5.   Once heated, arrange the kale leaves on a large baking sheet leaving ample space between them.

6.   Bake the leaves for 80 to 90 minutes flipping them once in between.

7.   Finally, allow them to cool completely and then store them in an air-tight container.

Green Salsa

Servings: 4

Cooking Time: 15 Minutes

Ingredients:

- 3 large heirloom tomatoes, chopped
- 1 green onion, finely chopped
- ½ bunch parsley, chopped
- 2 garlic cloves, minced
- 1 Jalapeño pepper, minced
- Juice of 1 lime
- ¼ cup olive oil Salt to taste
- Whole-grain tortilla chips

Directions:

1. Combine the tomatoes, green onion, parsley, garlic, jalapeño pepper, lime juice, olive oil, and salt in a bowl. Let it rest for minutes at room temperature. Serve with tortilla chips.

Kentucky Cauliflower with Mashed Parsnips

Servings: 6

Cooking Time: 35 Minutes

Ingredients:

- ½ cup unsweetened almond milk
- ¼ cup coconut flour
- ¼ tsp cayenne pepper
- ½ cup whole-grain breadcrumbs
- ½ cup grated plant-based mozzarella
- 30 oz cauliflower florets
- 1 lb parsnips, peeled and quartered
- 3 tbsp melted plant butter
- A pinch of nutmeg
- 1 tsp cumin powder
- 1 cup coconut cream
- 2 tbsp sesame oil

Directions:

1. Preheat oven to 425 F and line a baking sheet with parchment paper.

2. In a small bowl, combine almond milk, coconut flour, and cayenne pepper. In another bowl, mix salt,

breadcrumbs, and plant-based mozzarella cheese. Dip each cauliflower floret into the milk mixture, coating properly, and then into the cheese mixture. Place the breaded cauliflower on the baking sheet and bake in the oven for 30 minutes, turning once after 15 minutes.

3. Make slightly salted water in a saucepan and add the parsnips. Bring to boil over medium heat for 15 minutes or until the parsnips are fork tender. Drain and transfer to a bowl. Add in melted plant butter, cumin powder, nutmeg, and coconut cream. Puree the ingredients using an immersion blender until smooth. Spoon the parsnip mash into serving plates and drizzle with some sesame oil. Serve with the baked cauliflower when ready.

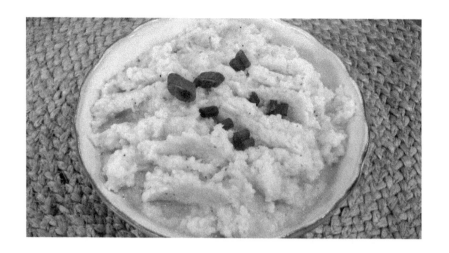

Pesto Zucchini Noodles

Servings: 4

Cooking Time: 0 Minutes

Ingredients:

- 4 little zucchini ends trimmed
- Cherry tomatoes
- 2 t. fresh lemon juice
- 1/3 c olive oil (best if extra-virgin)
- 2 cups packed basil leaves
- 2 c. garlic
- Salt and pepper to taste

Directions:

1. Spiral zucchini into noodles and set to the side.

2. In a food processor, combine the basil and garlic and chop. Slowly add olive oil while chopping. Then pulse blend it until thoroughly mixed.

3. In a big bowl, place the noodles and pour pesto sauce over the top. Toss to combine.

4. Garnish with tomatoes and serve and enjoy.

Mixed Vegetables with Basil

Servings: 4

Cooking Time: 40 Minutes

Ingredients:

- 2 medium zucchinis, chopped
- 2 medium yellow squash, chopped
- 1 red onion, cut into 1-inch wedges
- 1 red bell pepper, diced
- 1 cup cherry tomatoes, halved
- 4 tbsp olive oil
- Salt and black pepper to taste
- 3 garlic cloves, minced
- 2/3 cup whole-wheat breadcrumbs
- 1 lemon, zested
- ¼ cup chopped fresh basil

Directions:

1. Preheat the oven to 450 F and lightly grease a large baking sheet with cooking spray.

2. In a medium bowl, add the zucchini, yellow squash, red onion, bell pepper, tomatoes, olive oil, salt, black pepper, and garlic. Toss well and spread the mixture

53

on the baking sheet. Roast in the oven for to 30 minutes or until the vegetables are tender, while stirring every 5 minutes.

3. Meanwhile, heat the olive oil in a medium skillet and sauté the garlic until fragrant. Mix in the breadcrumbs, lemon zest, and basil. Cook for 2 to minutes. Remove the vegetables from the oven and toss in the breadcrumb's mixture. Serve warm.

Za'atar Roasted Zucchini Sticks

Servings: 5

Cooking Time: 1 Hour 35 Minutes

Ingredients:

- 1 ½ pounds zucchini, cut into sticks lengthwise
- 2 garlic cloves, crushed
- 2 tablespoons extra-virgin olive oil
- 1 teaspoon za'atar spice
- Kosher salt and ground black pepper, to taste

Directions:

1. Toss the zucchini with the remaining ingredients.

2. Lay the zucchini sticks in a single layer on a parchment-lined baking pan.

3. Bake at 2 degrees F for about 90 minutes until crisp and golden. Zucchini sticks will crisp up as they cool.

4. Bon appétit!

Nutrition Info: Per Serving: Calories: 85; Fat: 6.1g;

Carbs: 5.7g; Protein: 4.1g

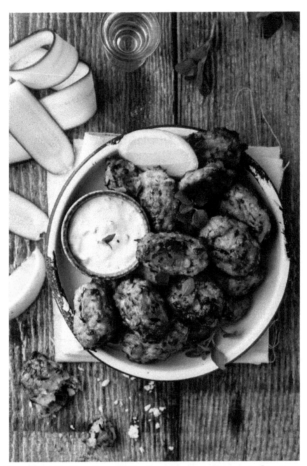

Tangy Fruit Salad with Lemon Dressing

Servings: 4

Cooking Time: 15 Minutes

Ingredients:

- Salad:
- ½ pound mixed berries
- ½ pound apples, cored and diced
- 8 ounces red grapes
- 2 kiwis, peeled and diced
- 2 large oranges, peeled and sliced
- 2 bananas, sliced
- Lemon Dressing:
- 2 tablespoons fresh lemon juice
- 1 teaspoon fresh ginger, peeled and minced
- 4 tablespoons agave syrup

Directions:

1. Mix all the ingredients for the salad until well combined.

2. Then, in a small mixing bowl, whisk all the lemon dressing ingredients.

3. Dress your salad and serve well chilled. Bon appétit!

Nutrition Info: Per Serving: Calories: 223; Fat: 0.8g; Carbs: 56.1g; Protein: 2.4g

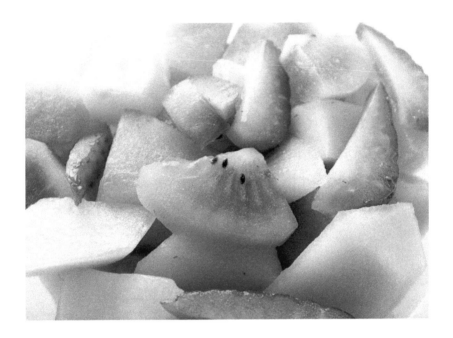

Nutty Date Cake

Servings: 4

Cooking Time: 1 Hour 30 Minutes

Ingredients:

- ½ cup cold plant butter, cut in pieces
- 1 tbsp flax seed powder
- ½ cup whole-wheat flour
- ¼ cup chopped pecans and walnuts
- 1 tsp baking powder
- 1 tsp baking soda
- 1 tsp cinnamon powder
- 1 tsp salt
- 1/3 cup pitted dates, chopped
- ½ cup pure date sugar
- 1 tsp vanilla extract
- ¼ cup pure date syrup for drizzling.

Directions:

1. Preheat oven to 350 F and lightly grease a round baking dish with some plant butter. In a small bowl, mix the flax seed powder with 3 tbsp water and allow thickening for 5 minutes to make the flax egg.

2.   In a food processor, add the flour, nuts, baking powder, baking soda, cinnamon powder, and salt. Blend until well combined. Add 1/3 cup of water, dates, date sugar, and vanilla. Process until smooth with tiny pieces of dates evident.

3.   Pour the batter into the baking dish and bake in the oven for 1 hour and 10 minutes or until a toothpick inserted comes out clean. Remove the dish from the oven, invert the cake onto a serving platter to cool, drizzle with the date syrup, slice, and serve.

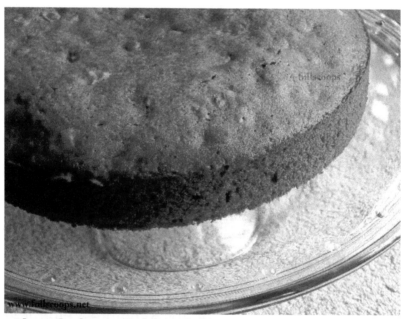

Tempting Quinoa Tabbouleh

Servings: 6

Cooking Time: 10 Minutes

Ingredients:

- 1 cup of well-rinsed quinoa

- 1 finely minced garlic clove

- ½ teaspoon of kosher salt

- ½ cup of extra virgin olive oil

- 2 tablespoons of fresh lemon juice
- Freshly ground black pepper
- 2 Persian cucumbers, cut into ¼-inch pieces
- 2 thinly sliced scallions
- 1 pint of halved cherry tomatoes
- ½ cup of chopped fresh mint
- 2/3 cup of chopped parsley

Directions:

1. Put a medium saucepan on high heat and boil the quinoa mixed with salt in ¼ cups of water. Decrease the heat to medium-low, cover the pot, and simmer everything until the quinoa is tender. The entire process will take 10 minutes. Remove the quinoa from heat and allow it to stand for 5 minutes. Fluff it with a fork.

2. In a small bowl, whisk the garlic with the lemon juice. Add the olive oil gradually. Mix the salt and pepper to taste.

3. On a baking sheet, spread the quinoa and allow it to cool. Shift it to a large bowl and mix ¼ of the dressing.

4. Add the tomatoes, scallions, herbs, and cucumber. Give them a good toss and season everything with pepper and salt. Add the remaining dressing.

Roasted Carrot and Bean Dip

Servings: 10

Cooking Time: 55 Minutes

Ingredients:

- 1 ½ pounds carrots, trimmed
- 2 tablespoons olive oil
- 4 tablespoons tahini
- 8 ounces canned cannellini beans, drained
- 1 teaspoon garlic, chopped
- 2 tablespoons lemon juice
- 2 tablespoons soy sauce
- Sea salt and ground black pepper, to taste
- 1/2 teaspoon paprika
- 1/2 teaspoon dried dill
- 1/4 cup pepitas, toasted

Directions:

1. Begin by preheating your oven to 390 degrees F. Line a roasting pan with parchment paper.

2. Now, toss the carrots with the olive oil and arrange them on the prepared roasting pan.

3. Roast the carrots for about 50 minutes or until tender. Transfer the roasted carrots to the bowl of your food processor.

4. Add in the tahini, beans, garlic, lemon juice, soy sauce, salt, black pepper, paprika and dill. Process until your dip is creamy and uniform.

5. Garnish with toasted pepitas and serve with dippers of choice. Bon appétit!

Nutrition Info: Per Serving: Calories: 121; Fat: 8.3g;

Carbs: 11.2g; Protein: 2.8g

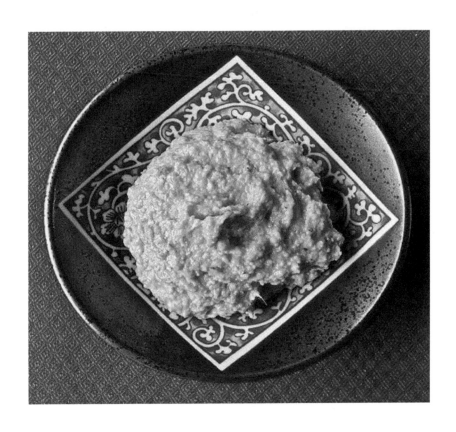

Pepita Cheese Tomato Chips

Servings: 6

Cooking Time: 15 Minutes

Ingredients:

- 5 tomatoes, sliced
- ¼ cup olive oil
- ½ cup pepitas seeds
- 1 tbsp nutritional yeast
- Salt and black pepper, to taste
- 1 tsp garlic puree

Directions:

1. Preheat oven to 400 F. Over the sliced tomatoes, drizzle olive oil. In a food processor, add pepitas seeds, nutritional yeast, garlic, salt, and pepper and pulse until the desired consistency is attained. Toss in tomato slices to coat. Set the tomato slices on a baking pan and bake for minutes.

Cinnamon Granola

Servings: 4

Cooking Time: 25 Minutes

Ingredients:

- 1 ½ t. cinnamon, ground
- 4 tbsp. maple syrup
- 1/5 oz. nuts
- 1 tbsp. chia seeds
- 5 tbsp. of the following:
- coconut flakes, unsweetened
- flaxseed meal

Directions:

1. Bring the oven to 350 heat setting.

2. In a medium mixing bowl, combine the flaxseed, coconut, chia seed, nuts, and maple syrup. Mix well until combined.

3. Line a cookie sheet with parchment and spread the mixture in a single layer on the cookie sheet.

4. Across the top, sprinkle the cinnamon.

5. Place the cookie sheet in the oven, and wait for 20 minutes, approximately.

6. Once done, take it out and allow the granola to cool while still on the sheet.

7. Once cool, crumble to your desired liking and enjoy.

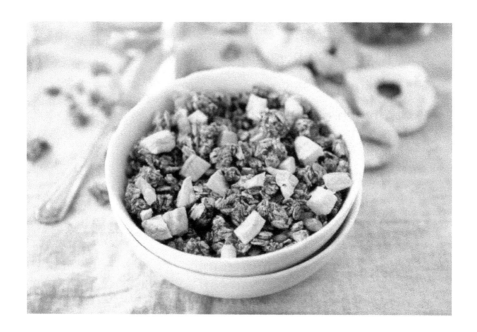

Old-fashioned Cookies

Servings: 12

Cooking Time: 45 Minutes

Ingredients:

*   1 cup all-purpose flour

*   1 teaspoon baking powder

*   A pinch of salt

*   A pinch of grated nutmeg

*   1/2 teaspoon ground cinnamon

*   1/4 teaspoon ground cardamom

*   1/2 cup peanut butter

*   2 tablespoons coconut oil, room temperature

*   2 tablespoons almond milk

*   1/2 cup brown sugar

*   1 teaspoon vanilla extract

*   1 cup vegan chocolate chips

Directions:

1.   In a mixing bowl, combine the flour, baking powder and spices.

2.   In another bowl, combine the peanut butter, coconut oil, almond milk, sugar and vanilla. Stir the wet

mixture into the dry ingredients and stir until well combined.

3.   Fold in the chocolate chips. Place the batter in your refrigerator for about minutes. Shape the batter into small cookies and arrange them on a parchment-lined cookie pan.

4.   Bake in the preheated oven at 350 degrees F for approximately 11 minutes. Transfer them to a wire rack to cool slightly before serving. Bon appétit!

Nutrition Info: Per Serving: Calories: 167; Fat: 8.6g;

Carbs: 19.6g; Protein: 2.7g

Dessert Crêpes
Servings: 10

Cooking Time: 10 Minutes

Ingredients:

- 1 ⅓ cups plain or vanilla soy milk
- 1 cup whole-grain flour
- ⅓ cup firm tofu, drained and crumbled
- 3 tablespoons vegan margarine, melted
- 2 tablespoons light brown sugar
- 1½ teaspoons pure vanilla extract
- ½teaspoon baking powder
- ⅛ teaspoon salt
- Canola or other neutral oil, for cooking

Directions:

1. Preparing the Ingredients

2. In a blender, combine all the ingredients (except the oil for cooking) and blend until smooth.

3. Heat a nonstick medium skillet or crêpe pan over medium-high heat. Coat the pan with a small amount of oil. Pour about tablespoons of the batter into the center of the skillet and tilt the pan to

spread the batter out thinly. Cook until golden on both sides, flipping once. Transfer to a platter and repeat with the remaining batter, oiling the pan as needed.

4. Finish and Serve

5. The crêpes can now be used in the recipes below or topped with your favorite dessert sauce or sautéed fruit. These taste best if used on the same day that they are made.

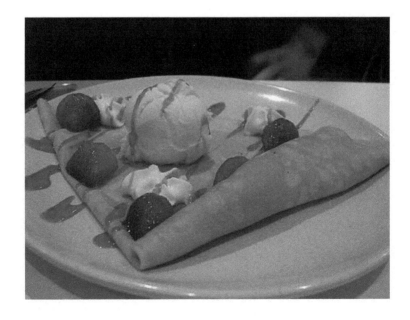

Baked Apples Filled with Nuts

Servings: 4

Cooking Time: 35 Minutes

Ingredients:

- 4 gala apples
- 3 tbsp pure maple syrup
- 4 tbsp almond flour
- 6 tbsp pure date sugar
- 6 tbsp plant butter, cold and cubed
- 1 cup chopped mixed nuts

Directions:

1. Preheat the oven the 400 F.

2. Slice off the top of the apples and use a melon baller or spoon to scoop out the cores of the apples. In a bowl, mix the maple syrup, almond flour, date sugar, butter, and nuts. Spoon the mixture into the apples and then bake in the oven for minutes or until the nuts are golden brown on top and the apples soft. Remove the apples from the oven, allow cooling, and serve.

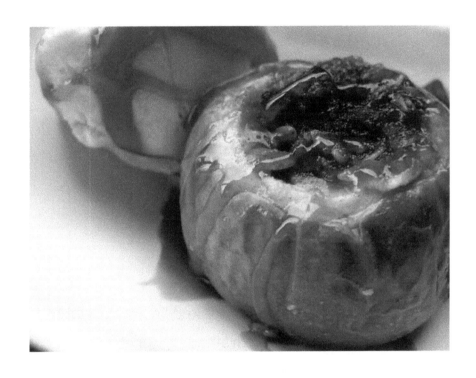

Chocolate Mint Grasshopper Pie

Servings: 4

Cooking Time: 0 Minute

Ingredients:

- For the Crust:
- 1 cup dates, soaked in warm water for 10 minutes in water, drained
- 1/8 teaspoons salt
- 1/2 cup pecans
- 1 teaspoons cinnamon
- 1/2 cup walnuts
- For the Filling:
- ½ cup mint leaves
- 2 cups of cashews, soaked in warm water for 10 minutes in water, drained
- 2 tablespoons coconut oil
- 1/4 cup and 2 tablespoons of agave
- 1/4 teaspoons spirulina
- 1/4 cup water

Directions:

1. Prepare the crust, and for this, place all its ingredients in a food processor and pulse for 3

76

to 5 minutes until the thick paste comes together.

2.   Take a 6-inch springform pan, grease it with oil, place crust mixture in it and spread and press the mixture evenly in the bottom and along the sides, and freeze until required.

3.   Prepare the filling and for this, place all its ingredients in a food processor, and pulse for 2 minutes until smooth.

4.   Pour the filling into prepared pan, smooth the top, and freeze for hours until set.

5.   Cut pie into slices and then serve.

Nutrition Info: Calories: 223.7 Cal; Fat: 7.5 g: Carbs:

36 g; Protein: 2.5 g; Fiber: 1 g

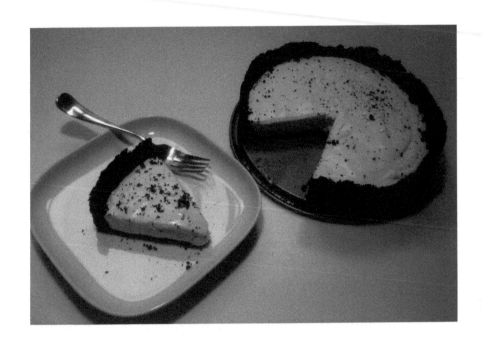

Date & Seed Bites

Servings: 10

Cooking Time: 0 Minutes

Ingredients:

- 1 cup cashew butter
- 6 Medjool dates, pitted
- 2/3 cup hemp seeds
- ¼ cup chia seeds
- ¼ cup unsweetened vegan protein powder
- ¾ cup unsweetened coconut, shredded

Directions:

1. In a food processor, place all the ingredients and pulse until well combined.

2. With your hands, make equal-sized balls from mixture.

3. In a shallow dish, place the coconut.

4. Roll the balls in the coconut evenly.

5. Refrigerate the balls till serving.

6. Arrange the balls onto a parchment paper-lined baking sheet in a single layer.

7. Refrigerate to set for about 30 minutes before serving.

Soy Chorizo & Avocado Tacos

Servings: 4

Cooking Time: 20 Minutes

Ingredients:

- 2 tbsp olive oil
- 8 oz soy chorizo
- 4 soft flour tortillas
- ¼ cup tofu mayonnaise
- 4 large lettuce leaves
- 2 ripe avocados, sliced
- 1 tomato, sliced

Directions:

1. Warm the oil in a skillet over medium heat. Place the soy chorizo and cook for 6 minutes on all sides, until browned. Set aside. Spread mayonnaise over tortillas and top with lettuce leaves and tomato siles. Cover with avocado slices and finish with soy chorizo. Roll up the tortillas and serve immediately.

Chocolate Campanelle with Hazelnuts

Servings: 4

Cooking Time: 10 Minutes

Ingredients:

- ½ cup chopped toasted hazelnuts
- ¼ cup vegan semisweet chocolate pieces
- 8 oz campanelle pasta
- 3 tbsp vegan margarine
- ¼ cup maple syrup

Directions:

1. Pulse the hazelnuts and chocolate pieces in a food processor until crumbly. Set aside.

2. Place the campanelle pasta in a pot with boiling salted water. Cook for 8-10 minutes until al dente, stirring often. Drain and back to the pot. Stir in almond butter and syrup and stir until the butter is melted. Remove to a plate and serve garnished with the chocolate-hazelnut mixture.

Waffles With Almond Flour

Servings: 4

Cooking Time: 15 Minutes

Ingredients:

- 1 cup almond milk
- 2 tbsps. chia seeds
- 2 tsp lemon juice
- 4 tbsps. coconut oil
- 1/2 cup almond flour
- 2 tbsps. maple syrup
- Cooking spray or cooking oil

Directions:

1. Mix coconut milk with lemon juice in a mixing bowl.

2. Leave it for 5-8 minutes on room temperature to turn it into butter milk.

3. Once coconut milk is turned into butter milk, add chai seeds into milk and whisk together.

4. Add other ingredients in milk mixture and mix well.

5. Preheat a waffle iron and spray it with coconut oil spray.

6. Pour 2 tbsp. of waffle mixture into the waffle machine and cook until golden.

7. Top with some berries and serve hot.

8. Enjoy with black coffee!

Nutrition Info: Protein: 5% 15 kcal Fat: 71% 199 kcal Carbohydrates: 23% 66 kcal

Vanilla Cranberry & Almond Balls

Servings: 12

Cooking Time: 25 Minutes

Ingredients:

- 2 tbsp almond butter
- 2 tbsp maple syrup
- ¾ cup cooked millet
- ¼ cup sesame seeds, toasted
- 1 tbsp chia seeds
- ½ tsp almond extract
- Zest of 1 orange
- 1 tbsp dried cranberries
- ¼ cup ground almonds

Directions:

1. Whisk the almond butter and syrup in a bowl, until creamy. Mix in millet, sesame seeds, chia seeds, almond extract, orange zest, cranberries, and almonds. Shape the mixture into balls and arrange on a parchment paper lined baking sheet. Let chill in the fridge for minutes.

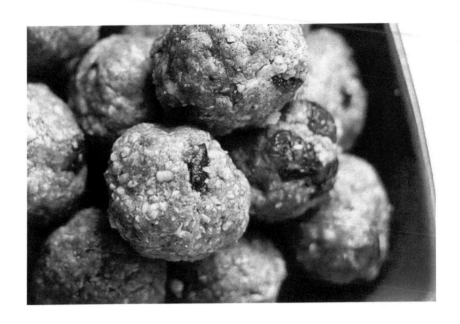

Cashew-chocolate Truffles

Servings: 12

Cooking Time: 0 Minutes

Ingredients:

- 1 cup raw cashews, soaked in water overnight
- ¾ cup pitted dates
- 2 tablespoons coconut oil
- 1 cup unsweetened shredded coconut, divided
- 1 to 2 tablespoons cocoa powder, to taste

Directions:

1. Preparing the Ingredients.

2. In a food processor, combine the cashews, dates, coconut oil, ½ cup of shredded coconut, and cocoa powder. Pulse until fully incorporated; it will resemble chunky cookie dough. Spread the remaining ½ cup of shredded coconut on a plate.

3. Form the mixture into tablespoon-size balls and roll on the plate to cover with the shredded coconut. Transfer to a parchment paper–lined

plate or baking sheet. Repeat to make 12 truffles.

4. Finish and Serve

5. Place the truffles in the refrigerator for 1 hour to set. Transfer the truffles to a storage container or freezer-safe bag and seal.

Nutrition Info: Per Serving: (1 truffle) Calories 238: Fat: 18g; Protein: 3g; Carbohydrates: 16g; Fiber: 4g; Sugar: 9g; Sodium: 9mg

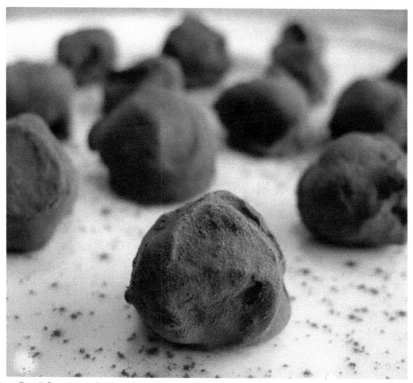

Tofu & Almond Pancakes

Servings: 10

Cooking Time: 15 Minutes

Ingredients:

- 1 ⅓ cups almond milk

- 1 cup almond flour

- ⅓ cup firm tofu, crumbled
- 3 tbsp plant butter, melted
- 2 tbsp pure date sugar
- 1 ½ tsp pure vanilla extract
- ½ tsp baking powder
- ⅛ tsp salt

Directions:

1. Blitz almond milk, tofu, butter, sugar, vanilla, baking powder, and salt in a blender until smooth. Heat a pan and coat with oil. Scoop a ladle of batter at the center and spread all over. Cook for 3-4 minutes until golden, turning once. Transfer to a plate and repeat the process until no batter is left. Serve.

Sweet Potato Toast

Servings: 1

Cooking Time: 10 Minutes

Ingredients:

- ½ of 1 Avocado, ripe
- 2 tbsp. Sun-dried Tomatoes
- 1 Sweet Potato, sliced into ¼-inch thick slices
- ½ cup Chickpeas
- Salt & Pepper, as needed
- 1 tsp. Lemon Juice
- Pinch of Red Pepper
- 2 tbsp. Vegan Cheese

Directions:

1. Start by slicing the sweet potato into five ¼ inch wide slices.

2. Next, toast the sweet potato in the toaster for 9 to 11 minutes.

3. Then, place the chickpeas in a medium-sized bowl and mash with the avocado.

4. Stir in the crushed red pepper, lemon juice, pepper, and salt.

5. Stir until everything comes together.

6. Finally, place the mixture on to the top of the sweet potato toast.

7. Top with cheese and sun-dried tomatoes.

Sesame Cabbage Sauté

Servings: 4

Cooking Time: 15 Minutes

Ingredients:

- 2 tbsp soy sauce
- 1 tbsp toasted sesame oil
- 1 tbsp hot sauce
- ½ tbsp pure date sugar
- ½ tbsp olive oil
- 1 head green cabbage, shredded
- 2 carrots, julienned
- 3 green onions, thinly sliced
- 2 garlic cloves, minced
- 1 tbsp fresh grated ginger
- Salt and black pepper to taste
- 1 tbsp sesame seeds

Directions:

1. In a small bowl, mix the soy sauce, sesame oil, hot sauce, and date sugar.

2. Heat the olive oil in a large skillet and sauté the cabbage, carrots, green onion, garlic, and ginger until

softened, 5 minutes. Mix in the prepared sauce and toss well. Cook for 1 to minutes. Dish the food and garnish with the sesame seeds.

Maple-pumpkin Cookies

Servings: 12

Cooking Time: 70 Minutes

Ingredients:

- 2-pound pumpkin, sliced
- 3 tbsp melted coconut oil, divided
- 1 tbsp maple syrup
- 1 cup whole-wheat flour
- 2 tsp baking powder Sea salt to taste

Directions:

1. Preheat oven to 360 F.

2. Place the pumpkin in a greased tray and bake for 45 minutes until tender. Let cool before mashing it.

3. Mix the mashed pumpkin, 1 ½ tbsp of coconut oil and maple syrup in a bowl.

4. Combine the flour and baking powder in another bowl. Fold in the pumpkin mixture and whisk with a fork until smooth.

5.   Divide the mixture into balls. Arrange spaced out on a lined with parchment paper baking sheet; flatten the balls until a cookie shape is formed. Brush with the remaining melted coconut oil. Bake for 10 minutes, until they rise and become gold. Serve cooled.

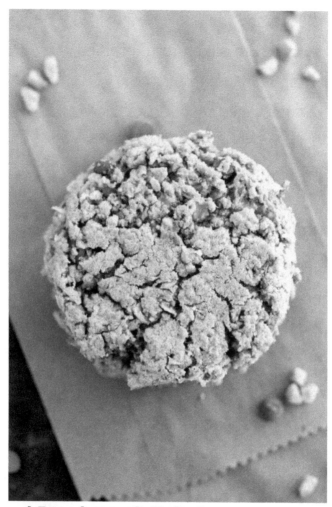

Layered Raspberry & Tofu Cups

Servings: 4

Cooking Time: 60 Minutes

Ingredients:

- ½ cup unsalted raw cashews

- 3 tbsp pure date sugar

- ½ cup soy milk

- ¾ cup firm silken tofu, drained

- 1 tsp vanilla extract

- 2 cups sliced raspberries

- 1 tsp fresh lemon juice

- Fresh mint leaves

Directions:

1. Grind the cashews and 3 tbsp of date sugar, in a blender until a fine powder is obtained. Pour in soy milk and blitz until smooth. Add in tofu and vanilla and pulse until creamy. Remove to a bowl and refrigerate covered for 30 minutes.

2. In a bowl, mix the raspberries, lemon juice and remaining date sugar. Let sit for minutes. Assemble by alternating into small cups one layer of raspberries and one layer of cashew cream, ending with the cashew cream. Serve garnished with mint leaves.

Full-flavored Vanilla Ice Cream

Servings: 8

Cooking Time: 20 Minutes

Ingredients:

- 1 1/2 cups canned coconut milk
- 1 cup coconut whipping cream
- 1 frozen banana cut into chunks
- 1 cup vanilla sugar
- 3 Tbsp apple sauce
- 2 tsp pure vanilla extract
- 1 tsp Xanthan gum or agar-agar thickening agent

Directions:

1. Add all ingredients in a food processor; process until all ingredients combined well.

2. Place the ice cream mixture in a freezer-safe container with a lid over.

3. Freeze for at least 4 hours.

4. Remove frozen mixture to a bowl and beat with a mixer to break up the ice crystals.

5. Repeat this process 3 to 4 times.

6.   Let the ice cream at room temperature for 15 minutes before serving.

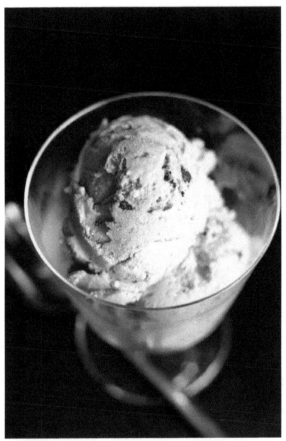

Country-style Apricot Dump Cake

Servings: 8

Cooking Time: 10 Minutes

Ingredients:

- 10 apricots, pitted and halved
- 1 tablespoon crystallized ginger
- 1/4 cup brown sugar
- 1 cup all-purpose flour
- 1 teaspoon baking powder
- 1/2 teaspoon ground cinnamon
- 4 tablespoons agave syrup
- A pinch of kosher salt
- A pinch of grated nutmeg
- 1/4 cup coconut oil, room temperature
- 1/2 cup almond milk

Directions:

1. Arrange the apricots on the bottom of a lightly oiled baking pan. Sprinkle ginger and brown sugar over them.

2. In a mixing bowl, thoroughly combine the flour, baking powder, cinnamon, agave syrup, salt and nutmeg.

3. Add in the coconut oil and almond milk and mix until everything is well incorporated. Spread the topping mixture over the fruit layer.

4.   Bake your cake at 360 degrees F for about minutes or until the top is golden brown. Bon appétit!

Nutrition Info: Per Serving: Calories: 226; Fat: 7.5g; Carbs: 38.8g; Protein: 2.4g

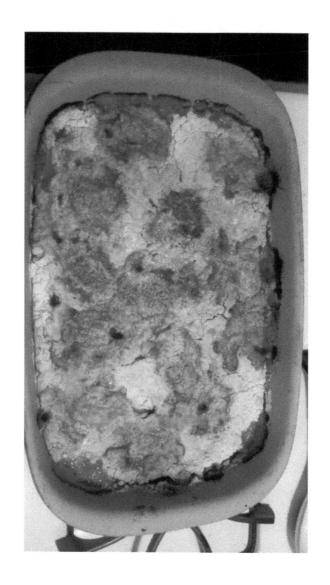

Sherry-lime Mango Dessert

Servings: 4

Cooking Time: 15 Minutes

Ingredients:

- 3 ripe mangoes, cubed
- ⅓ cup pure date sugar
- 2 tbsp fresh lime juice
- ½ cup Sherry
- Fresh mint sprigs

Directions:

1. Arrange the mango cubes on a baking sheet. Sprinkle with some date and let sit covered for 30 minutes. Sprinkle with lime juice and sherry. Refrigerate covered for hour. Remove from the fridge and let sit for a few minutes at room temperature. Serve in glasses topped with mint.

Chocolate Cookies

Servings: 4

Cooking Time: 5 Minutes

Ingredients:

- 1/2 cup coconut oil
- 1 cup agave syrup
- 1/2 cup cocoa powder
- 1/2 teaspoon salt
- 2 cups peanuts, chopped
- 1 cup peanut butter
- 2 cups sunflower seeds

Directions:

1. Take a small saucepan, place it over medium heat, add the first three ingredients, and cook for 3 minutes until melted.

2. Boil the mixture for 1 minute, then remove the pan from heat and stir in salt and butter until smooth.

3. Fold in nuts and seeds until combined, then drop the mixture in the form of molds onto the baking

sheet lined with wax paper and refrigerate for minutes.

4.   Serve straight away.

Nutrition Info: Calories: 148 Cal; Fat: 7.4 g: Carbs: 20 g; Protein: 1.5 g; Fiber: 0.6 g

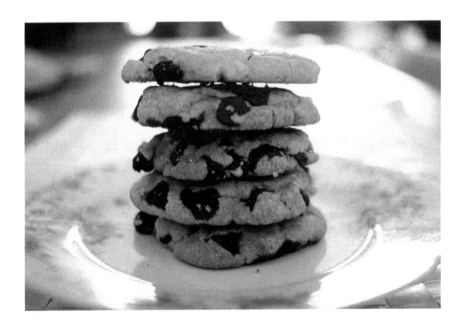

Mango Coconut Cheesecake

Servings: 4

Cooking Time: 0 Minute

Ingredients:

- For the Crust:
- 1 cup macadamia nuts
- 1 cup dates, pitted, soaked in hot water for 10 minutes
- For the Filling:
- 2 cups cashews, soaked in warm water for 10 minutes
- 1/2 cup and 1 tablespoon maple syrup
- 1/3 cup and 2 tablespoons coconut oil
- 1/4 cup lemon juice
- 1/2 cup and 2 tablespoons coconut milk, unsweetened, chilled
- For the Topping:
- 1 cup fresh mango slices

Directions:

1. Prepare the crust, and for this, place nuts in a food processor and process until mixture resembles crumbs.

2. Drain the dates, add them to the food processor and blend for minutes until thick mixture comes together.

3. Take a 4-inch cheesecake pan, place date mixture in it, spread and press evenly, and set aside.

4. Prepare the filling and for this, place all its ingredients in a food processor and blend for 3 minutes until smooth.

5. Pour the filling into the crust, spread evenly, and then freeze for 4 hours until set.

6. Top the cake with mango slices and then serve.

Nutrition Info: Calories: 200 Cal; Fat: 11 g: Carbs: 22.5 g; Protein: 2 g; Fiber: 1 g

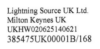

9 781803 171463